Moon Diet

Transform Your Body and Mind with the Moon's Natural Rhythm

Marc Ben

Obey Life Publishing

To my wife Filomena

Acknowledgments

As we reach the conclusion of the "Moon Diet" journey, I want to extend my deepest gratitude to all the collaborators, nutritionists, and chefs from Brazil who have played an instrumental role in shaping this dietary guide. Your expertise, dedication, and passion for healthy living have been invaluable.

Brazil's culinary heritage is renowned not only for its vibrant flavors but also for its deep-rooted commitment to nutritious, wholesome food. I would also like to emphasize the importance of considering individual dietary needs and restrictions when following the recipes and advice provided in this book. Each person's body is unique, and what works for one may not work for another. It is crucial to be mindful of potential food allergies, intolerances, and other dietary restrictions that may affect your health. I strongly recommend consulting with a healthcare professional or a registered dietitian before making any significant changes to your diet.

Thank you once again to everyone who contributed to this project. Your support has made this journey not only possible but deeply enriching.

Table of Content

Acknowledgments 3

Table of Content 4

Introduction 6

Moon Phases and Diet.. 8

More About the Moon Diet (Lunar Fast) 12

Week Moon Diet Plan.. 16

Week 1: New Moon Phase 18

Week 2: Waxing Crescent Moon................................. 25

Week 3: Full Moon... 32

Week 4: Waning Crescent Moon................................. 40

SECOND OPTION LIST 48

Week 1: New Moon Phase 48

Week 2: Waxing Crescent Moon................................. 56

Week 3: Full Moon... 64

Week 4: Waning Crescent Moon 71

EXTRA – NUTS, the best part!!........................79

Here's a list of foods, snacks, and drinks to avoid
during the 4-week "Moon Diet" period to help you stay
on track with your goals. 86

Physical Activities:..91

Mindfulness and Relaxation:..........................93

Sleep and Recovery:......................................95

Hydration and Detox:....................................96

Lifestyle Adjustments: 97

Stress Management: 98

Artists and Composers:..................................99

Places to Find Meditation and Relaxation Music: 102

Finding the Next Lunar Phases Online 110

Introduction

Presentation of the Moon Diet Concept

The "Moon Diet" is a unique approach to healthy eating based on the phases of the moon. Just as the moon influences the tides, it is believed to affect our bodies and health as well. This diet aims to harmonize our eating habits with the lunar cycle, promoting detoxification, energy, fullness, and relaxation according to each phase of the moon. By following the Moon Diet, you can enjoy a balanced diet and a healthier, more harmonious lifestyle.

The Influence of the Moon Phases on Diet and Health

Since ancient times, the moon has been a source of mystery and fascination for humanity. Various cultures believe that the moon phases can influence plant growth, ocean tides, and even human behavior. The Moon Diet is based on the idea that by synchronizing our eating habits with the moon phases, we can enhance the benefits for our health. During the new moon, our body is more receptive to detoxification, while during the waxing moon, we need more energy and nutrients. The full moon invites us to fullness and satisfaction, and the waning moon is ideal for relaxation and cleansing.

How to Use This Manual

This manual is organized to facilitate your journey with the Moon Diet. Each week is aligned with a moon phase and includes options for breakfast, lunch, afternoon snack, and dinner, with two options for each meal. The recipes are designed to be simple, accessible, and affordable, using ingredients that are easy to find. Follow the 4-week plan and try the recipes as recommended to maximize the benefits of each lunar phase.

Moon Phases and Diet

New Moon: Renewal and Detoxification

Recommended Foods:

Dark leafy greens (kale, spinach)

Citrus fruits (lemon, orange)

Cruciferous vegetables (broccoli, cauliflower)

Detox teas (green tea, dandelion tea)

Fiber-rich foods (oats, quinoa)

Description:

The new moon is the ideal time to start a detoxification and body renewal process. During this phase, the body is more prepared to eliminate toxins and regenerate. Fiber-rich and antioxidant-rich foods help cleanse the digestive system and improve liver function. Detox teas and lemon water are also recommended to aid the detoxification process.

Waxing Moon: Energy and Growth

Recommended Foods:

Lean proteins (chicken, fish, tofu)

Whole grains (brown rice, quinoa)

Legumes (beans, lentils)

Vitamin-rich fruits (mango, pineapple)

Nuts (almonds, walnuts)

Description:

During the waxing moon phase, the body needs more energy and nutrients to support growth and development. Protein-rich foods and whole grains provide the necessary energy for daily activities. Legumes and nuts are sources of essential vitamins and minerals for health. During this phase, it is important to consume balanced meals that provide sustained energy.

Full Moon: Plenitude and Satisfaction

Recommended Foods:

Complex carbohydrates (sweet potato, pumpkin)

Colorful fruits and vegetables (beetroot, carrot, strawberry)

Light dairy (yogurt, cottage cheese)

Whole foods (whole grain bread, oats)

Superfoods (chia, flaxseed)

Description:

The full moon is a phase of fullness and satisfaction, where the body seeks foods that provide a sense of satiety and pleasure. Complex carbohydrates and whole foods help maintain energy and a sense of well-being. Colorful fruits and vegetables are rich in antioxidants and fibers, promoting healthy digestion. Superfoods like chia and flaxseed can be added to meals to increase nutritional value.

Waning Moon: Cleansing and Relaxation

Recommended Foods:

Light soups and broths

Leafy vegetables (lettuce, arugula)

Low-calorie fruits (melon, strawberry)

Calming teas (chamomile, lemon balm)

Fermented foods (yogurt, kefir)

Description:

The waning moon phase is a period of cleansing and relaxation, ideal for relieving stress and preparing the body for a new cycle. Light soups and broths are easy to digest and help with hydration. Leafy vegetables and low-calorie fruits provide essential nutrients without overloading the digestive system. Calming teas and fermented foods promote gut health and general well-being.

More About the Moon Diet (Lunar Fast)

History and Origin

The Moon Diet, also known as the Lunar Fast, has roots in ancient practices and beliefs that align human activities with lunar cycles. This diet is based on the idea that the moon, which influences the tides, also affects the water content in our bodies, which is roughly 60% water. Different phases of the moon are thought to have varying effects on our body's detoxification processes, metabolism, and overall well-being.

Principles of the Moon Diet

Lunar Influence: The diet leverages the moon's phases to optimize bodily functions. The belief is that during certain phases, the body is more efficient in detoxifying, absorbing nutrients, and maintaining energy levels.

Cleansing and Fasting: The diet often involves fasting or cleansing, particularly during the new moon and full moon phases, when the body's detoxification processes are believed to be at their peak.

Phases and Diet Plan:

New Moon: A time for detoxification. It is recommended to drink plenty of water and herbal teas, and consume light, easy-to-digest foods. Some followers of the Moon Diet may also choose to fast during this phase.

Waxing Moon: This phase focuses on building energy and strength. The diet includes nutrient-dense foods like proteins, whole grains, and legumes to support growth and energy accumulation.

Full Moon: During the full moon, the body's absorption capacity is at its highest. It's a time to enjoy wholesome, nutrient-rich foods and maintain a balanced diet. Some people may also choose to fast or detox during the full moon to enhance the body's cleansing processes.

Waning Moon: This is a phase of relaxation and cleansing. The focus is on light, easily digestible foods, and calming teas that aid in relaxation and preparing the body for the next cycle.

Benefits of the Moon Diet

Enhanced Detoxification: Aligning with the new moon and full moon phases can help maximize the body's natural detoxification processes, potentially leading to better elimination of toxins.

Improved Digestion: By consuming lighter foods during the new moon and waning moon phases, you may give your digestive system a break, leading to improved digestion and gut health.

Balanced Energy Levels: The waxing moon phase encourages the intake of nutrient-dense foods that provide sustained energy, helping to avoid energy slumps.

Mindfulness and Rhythm: Following the lunar phases can bring a sense of rhythm and mindfulness to your eating habits, encouraging a more thoughtful approach to nutrition and overall well-being.

Practical Tips for the Moon Diet

Hydration: Regardless of the phase, staying hydrated is crucial. Drink plenty of water and herbal teas, especially during detox phases.

Natural and Whole Foods: Focus on consuming natural, whole foods that are minimally processed. This includes fresh fruits, vegetables, whole grains, lean proteins, and healthy fats.

Listen to Your Body: Pay attention to how your body responds to different foods and phases. Adjust your diet accordingly to meet your personal needs and preferences.

Plan: Use the lunar calendar to plan your meals and fasting days in advance. This will help you stay organized and committed to the diet. Directions to find lunar calendar, please see last page.

Gentle Exercise: Incorporate gentle exercise like yoga, walking, or stretching into your routine, especially during the waning moon phase to promote relaxation and overall health.

Week Moon Diet Plan

Week 1: New Moon

Focus on detoxifying foods like leafy greens, citrus fruits, and herbal teas.

Consider a one-day fast or consume only liquids like smoothies and broths.

Week 2: Waxing Moon

Incorporate energy-building foods such as lean proteins, whole grains, and legumes.

Maintain a balanced diet with nutrient-dense meals.

Week 3: Full Moon

Enjoy a variety of wholesome, nutrient-rich foods.

Consider a one-day fast or light detox to enhance the body's natural cleansing processes.

Week 4: Waning Moon

Focus on light, easily digestible foods like soups, broths, and leafy vegetables.

Drink calming teas to aid in relaxation and prepare the body for the next cycle.

Conclusion

The Moon Diet offers a holistic approach to nutrition that aligns with the natural rhythms of the lunar cycle. By following the Moon Diet, you may experience enhanced detoxification, improved digestion, balanced energy levels, and a more mindful approach to eating. Whether you choose to follow the diet strictly or adapt it to your needs, the principles of the Moon Diet can provide a framework for a healthier and more harmonious lifestyle.

Week 1: New Moon Phase

Focus: Cleansing and detoxifying the body

Day 1:

- **Breakfast:**

  - **Option 1:** Green Smoothie (Spinach, Banana, Water, and Chia Seeds)

  - **Option 2:** Oatmeal with Honey and Sliced Almonds

- **Lunch:**

  - **Option 1:** Lentil Soup with Carrots and Celery

  - **Option 2:** Quinoa Salad with Cucumber, Tomatoes, and Lemon Dressing

- **Snack:**

  - **Option 1:** Apple Slices with Peanut Butter

  - **Option 2:** Carrot Sticks with Hummus

- **Dinner:**

  - o **Option 1:** Grilled Chicken with Steamed Broccoli and Brown Rice

  - o **Option 2:** Baked Salmon with Mixed Greens and Sweet Potato

Day 2:

- **Breakfast:**

  - o **Option 1:** Yogurt with Granola and Mixed Berries

  - o **Option 2:** Scrambled Eggs with Whole Grain Toast

- **Lunch:**

  - o **Option 1:** Spinach and Chickpea Salad with Olive Oil Dressing

  - o **Option 2:** Vegetable Stir-fry with Tofu and Brown Rice

- **Snack:**

  - o **Option 1:** Handful of Mixed Nuts

  - o **Option 2:** Smoothie (Mango, Pineapple, and Coconut Water)

- **Dinner:**

  - o **Option 1:** Baked Tilapia with Garlic and Lemon, served with Asparagus

  - o **Option 2:** Turkey Lettuce Wraps with Avocado and Salsa

Day 3:

- **Breakfast:**

  - o **Option 1:** Smoothie Bowl with Banana, Blueberries, and Flaxseeds

  - o **Option 2:** Whole Grain Pancakes with Honey and Fresh Berries

- **Lunch:**

  - o **Option 1:** Tomato and Basil Soup with Whole Grain Crackers

  - o **Option 2:** Grilled Vegetable Wrap with Hummus

- **Snack:**

  - o **Option 1:** Sliced Cucumber with Cottage Cheese

  - o **Option 2:** Pear with Almond Butter

- **Dinner:**

    - o **Option 1:** Chicken and Vegetable Skewers with Quinoa

    - o **Option 2:** Zucchini Noodles with Marinara Sauce and Grilled Shrimp

Day 4:

- **Breakfast:**

    - o **Option 1:** Avocado Toast with a Poached Egg

    - o **Option 2:** Smoothie (Kale, Pineapple, and Almond Milk)

- **Lunch:**

    - o **Option 1:** Beet and Goat Cheese Salad with Walnuts

    - o **Option 2:** Quinoa Bowl with Black Beans, Corn, and Avocado

- **Snack:**

    - o **Option 1:** Rice Cakes with Hummus and Sliced Tomatoes

    - o **Option 2:** Smoothie (Strawberries, Banana, and Almond Milk)

- **Dinner:**

  - o **Option 1:** Grilled Turkey Burgers with Sweet Potato Fries

  - o **Option 2:** Baked Cod with Lemon, Garlic, and a Side of Green Beans

Day 5:

- **Breakfast:**

  - o **Option 1:** Chia Pudding with Mixed Berries

  - o **Option 2:** Whole Grain Cereal with Almond Milk and Sliced Bananas

- **Lunch:**

  - o **Option 1:** Greek Salad with Grilled Chicken

  - o **Option 2:** Black Bean Soup with a Side of Cornbread

- **Snack:**

  - o **Option 1:** Mixed Fruit Salad

  - o **Option 2:** Sliced Bell Peppers with Guacamole

- **Dinner:**

  - o **Option 1:** Stuffed Peppers with Ground Turkey and Quinoa

  - o **Option 2:** Grilled Eggplant with Tomato and Basil

Day 6:

- **Breakfast:**

  - o **Option 1:** Smoothie (Spinach, Mango, and Coconut Water)

  - o **Option 2:** Greek Yogurt with Honey and Walnuts

- **Lunch:**

  - o **Option 1:** Caprese Salad with a Drizzle of Balsamic Vinegar

  - o **Option 2:** Lentil Salad with Cucumber, Tomatoes, and Feta

- **Snack:**

  - o **Option 1:** Almonds and Dried Cranberries

  - o **Option 2:** Apple Slices with Cinnamon

- **Dinner:**

    - o **Option 1:** Grilled Chicken with Roasted Brussels Sprouts

    - o **Option 2:** Baked Fish with Mixed Vegetables and Quinoa

Day 7:

- **Breakfast:**

    - o **Option 1:** Smoothie (Blueberries, Banana, Spinach, and Almond Milk)

    - o **Option 2:** Overnight Oats with Almond Butter and Chia Seeds

- **Lunch:**

    - o **Option 1:** Avocado and Cucumber Sushi Rolls

    - o **Option 2:** Tomato Basil Quinoa with Grilled Chicken

- **Snack:**

    - o **Option 1:** Celery Sticks with Almond Butter

    - o **Option 2:** Berry Smoothie (Raspberries, Strawberries, and Greek Yogurt)

- **Dinner:**

  - o **Option 1:** Grilled Salmon with Steamed Broccoli

  - o **Option 2:** Vegetable Stir-Fry with Brown Rice

Week 2: Waxing Crescent Moon

Focus: Building and nourishing the body

Day 8:

- **Breakfast:**

  - o **Option 1:** Scrambled Eggs with Spinach and Whole Grain Toast

  - o **Option 2:** Smoothie (Banana, Almond Butter, and Oats)

- **Lunch:**

  - o **Option 1:** Grilled Chicken Caesar Salad with a Light Dressing

  - o **Option 2:** Chickpea and Avocado Salad with Lemon Dressing

- **Snack:**

  - o **Option 1:** Hard-Boiled Egg with a Sprinkle of Paprika

  - o **Option 2:** Handful of Trail Mix (Nuts, Seeds, and Dried Fruits)

- **Dinner:**

  - o **Option 1:** Grilled Steak with Mashed Sweet Potatoes and Steamed Broccoli

  - o **Option 2:** Baked Chicken with Quinoa and Roasted Vegetables

Day 9:

- **Breakfast:**

  - o **Option 1:** Greek Yogurt with Honey, Granola, and Mixed Berries

  - o **Option 2:** Oatmeal with Almonds and Dried Cranberries

- **Lunch:**

  - o **Option 1:** Tuna Salad with Whole Grain Crackers

  - o **Option 2:** Quinoa Bowl with Black Beans, Corn, and Avocado

- **Snack:**

    - o **Option 1:** Apple Slices with Peanut Butter

    - o **Option 2:** Smoothie (Spinach, Mango, and Coconut Water)

- **Dinner:**

    - o **Option 1:** Grilled Shrimp with Zucchini Noodles and Pesto

    - o **Option 2:** Turkey Meatballs with Marinara Sauce and Whole Grain Pasta

Day 10:

- **Breakfast:**

    - o **Option 1:** Whole Grain Pancakes with Honey and Sliced Bananas

    - o **Option 2:** Smoothie (Mixed Berries, Greek Yogurt, and Oats)

- **Lunch:**

    - o **Option 1:** Quinoa Salad with Roasted Vegetables and Feta

    - o **Option 2:** Lentil Soup with Whole Grain Bread

- **Snack:**

  - o **Option 1:** Carrot Sticks with Hummus

  - o **Option 2:** Mixed Fruit Salad

- **Dinner:**

  - o **Option 1:** Grilled Chicken Breast with Brown Rice and Steamed Green Beans

  - o **Option 2:** Baked Cod with Garlic, Lemon, and a Side of Asparagus

Day 11:

- **Breakfast:**

  - o **Option 1:** Avocado Toast with a Poached Egg

  - o **Option 2:** Smoothie (Kale, Pineapple, and Almond Milk)

- **Lunch:**

  - o **Option 1:** Spinach and Quinoa Salad with Lemon Dressing

  - o **Option 2:** Turkey Wrap with Avocado and Tomato

- **Snack:**

    - o **Option 1:** Handful of Mixed Nuts

    - o **Option 2:** Sliced Cucumber with Cottage Cheese

- **Dinner:**

    - o **Option 1:** Baked Salmon with Sweet Potato Fries and a Side Salad

    - o **Option 2:** Grilled Tofu with Stir-Fried Vegetables and Brown Rice

Day 12:

- **Breakfast:**

    - o **Option 1:** Chia Pudding with Mixed Berries

    - o **Option 2:** Scrambled Eggs with Spinach and Whole Grain Toast

- **Lunch:**

    - o **Option 1:** Grilled Chicken Caesar Salad with a Light Dressing

    - o **Option 2:** Lentil Salad with Cucumber, Tomatoes, and Feta

- **Snack:**

  - o **Option 1:** Celery Sticks with Almond Butter

  - o **Option 2:** Smoothie (Strawberries, Banana, and Almond Milk)

- **Dinner:**

  - o **Option 1:** Grilled Turkey Burgers with Sweet Potato Fries

  - o **Option 2:** Stuffed Peppers with Ground Turkey and Quinoa

Day 13:

- **Breakfast:**

  - o **Option 1:** Smoothie (Spinach, Banana, and Almond Milk)

  - o **Option 2:** Whole Grain Cereal with Almond Milk and Sliced Bananas

- **Lunch:**

  - o **Option 1:** Black Bean Soup with a Side of Cornbread

  - o **Option 2:** Greek Salad with Grilled Chicken

- **Snack:**

  - o **Option 1:** Rice Cakes with Hummus and Sliced Tomatoes

  - o **Option 2:** Sliced Bell Peppers with Guacamole

- **Dinner:**

  - o **Option 1:** Grilled Chicken with Roasted Brussels Sprouts

  - o **Option 2:** Zucchini Noodles with Marinara Sauce and Grilled Shrimp

Day 14:

- **Breakfast:**

  - o **Option 1:** Smoothie (Blueberries, Banana, Spinach, and Almond Milk)

  - o **Option 2:** Greek Yogurt with Honey and Walnuts

- **Lunch:**

  - o **Option 1:** Avocado and Cucumber Sushi Rolls

  - o **Option 2:** Caprese Salad with a Drizzle of Balsamic Vinegar

- **Snack:**

    - o **Option 1:** Almonds and Dried Cranberries

    - o **Option 2:** Mixed Fruit Salad

- **Dinner:**

    - o **Option 1:** Grilled Salmon with Steamed Broccoli

    - o **Option 2:** Grilled Steak with Mashed Sweet Potatoes and Steamed Broccoli

---

Week 3: Full Moon

Focus: Energy and activity, more substantial meals

Day 15:

- **Breakfast:**

    - o **Option 1:** Whole Grain Pancakes with Maple Syrup and Fresh Berries

    - o **Option 2:** Scrambled Eggs with Avocado and Whole Grain Toast

- **Lunch:**

  - o **Option 1:** Quinoa Salad with Roasted Vegetables and Feta

  - o **Option 2:** Tuna Salad with Whole Grain Crackers

- **Snack:**

  - o **Option 1:** Greek Yogurt with Honey and Almonds

  - o **Option 2:** Smoothie (Mixed Berries, Greek Yogurt, and Oats)

- **Dinner:**

  - o **Option 1:** Grilled Chicken Breast with Brown Rice and Steamed Green Beans

  - o **Option 2:** Baked Cod with Garlic, Lemon, and Asparagus

Day 16:

- **Breakfast:**

  - o **Option 1:** Oatmeal with Almond Butter, Chia Seeds, and Sliced Bananas

  - o **Option 2:** Smoothie (Kale, Pineapple, and Coconut Water)

- **Lunch:**

    - o **Option 1:** Grilled Vegetable Wrap with Hummus

    - o **Option 2:** Tomato Basil Soup with Whole Grain Bread

- **Snack:**

    - o **Option 1:** Apple Slices with Peanut Butter

    - o **Option 2:** Handful of Trail Mix (Nuts, Seeds, and Dried Fruits)

- **Dinner:**

    - o **Option 1:** Baked Salmon with Sweet Potato Fries and a Side Salad

    - o **Option 2:** Grilled Tofu with Stir-Fried Vegetables and Brown Rice

Day 17:

- **Breakfast:**

    - o **Option 1:** Smoothie Bowl with Banana, Blueberries, and Flaxseeds

    - o **Option 2:** Scrambled Eggs with Spinach and Whole Grain Toast

- **Lunch:**

  - o **Option 1:** Greek Salad with Grilled Chicken

  - o **Option 2:** Black Bean Soup with a Side of Cornbread

- **Snack:**

  - o **Option 1:** Sliced Bell Peppers with Guacamole

  - o **Option 2:** Mixed Fruit Salad

- **Dinner:**

  - o **Option 1:** Grilled Turkey Burgers with Sweet Potato Fries

  - o **Option 2:** Zucchini Noodles with Marinara Sauce and Grilled Shrimp

Day 18:

- **Breakfast:**

  - o **Option 1:** Chia Pudding with Mixed Berries

  - o **Option 2:** Whole Grain Pancakes with Maple Syrup and Fresh Berries

- **Lunch:**

  - o **Option 1:** Caprese Salad with a Drizzle of Balsamic Vinegar

  - o **Option 2:** Lentil Salad with Cucumber, Tomatoes, and Feta

- **Snack:**

  - o **Option 1:** Rice Cakes with Hummus and Sliced Tomatoes

  - o **Option 2:** Sliced Cucumber with Cottage Cheese

- **Dinner:**

  - o **Option 1:** Grilled Chicken Breast with Quinoa and Roasted Vegetables

  - o **Option 2:** Grilled Steak with Mashed Sweet Potatoes and Steamed Broccoli

Day 19:

- **Breakfast:**

    - **Option 1:** Greek Yogurt with Honey, Granola, and Mixed Berries

    - **Option 2:** Smoothie (Spinach, Banana, and Almond Milk)

- **Lunch:**

    - **Option 1:** Avocado and Cucumber Sushi Rolls

    - **Option 2:** Quinoa Salad with Roasted Vegetables and Feta

- **Snack:**

    - **Option 1:** Apple Slices with Almond Butter

    - **Option 2:** Mixed Fruit Salad

- **Dinner:**

    - **Option 1:** Grilled Shrimp with Zucchini Noodles and Pesto

    - **Option 2:** Turkey Meatballs with Marinara Sauce and Whole Grain Pasta

Day 20:

- **Breakfast:**

    - **Option 1:** Smoothie (Kale, Mango, and Coconut Water)

    - **Option 2:** Overnight Oats with Almond Butter and Chia Seeds

- **Lunch:**

    - **Option 1:** Tuna Salad with Whole Grain Crackers

    - **Option 2:** Spinach and Quinoa Salad with Lemon Dressing

- **Snack:**

    - **Option 1:** Handful of Mixed Nuts

    - **Option 2:** Celery Sticks with Almond Butter

- **Dinner:**

    - **Option 1:** Baked Tilapia with Garlic and Lemon, served with Asparagus

    - **Option 2:** Grilled Chicken with Roasted Brussels Sprouts

Day 21:

- **Breakfast:**

    - o **Option 1:** Whole Grain Cereal with Almond Milk and Sliced Bananas

    - o **Option 2:** Smoothie (Blueberries, Banana, Spinach, and Almond Milk)

- **Lunch:**

    - o **Option 1:** Chickpea and Avocado Salad with Lemon Dressing

    - o **Option 2:** Tomato Basil Soup with Whole Grain Crackers

- **Snack:**

    - o **Option 1:** Hard-Boiled Egg with a Sprinkle of Paprika

    - o **Option 2:** Almonds and Dried Cranberries

- **Dinner:**

    - o **Option 1:** Grilled Steak with Quinoa and Roasted Vegetables

    - o **Option 2:** Stuffed Peppers with Ground Turkey and Quinoa

Week 4: Waning Crescent Moon

Focus: Preparing for the next cycle, lighter meals

Day 22:

- **Breakfast:**

    o **Option 1:** Chia Pudding with Mixed Berries

    o **Option 2:** Greek Yogurt with Honey and Walnuts

- **Lunch:**

    o **Option 1:** Caprese Salad with a Drizzle of Balsamic Vinegar

    o **Option 2:** Spinach and Quinoa Salad with Lemon Dressing

- **Snack:**

    o **Option 1:** Sliced Bell Peppers with Guacamole

    o **Option 2:** Mixed Fruit Salad

- **Dinner:**

    - o **Option 1:** Baked Cod with Garlic, Lemon, and a Side of Asparagus

    - o **Option 2:** Grilled Tofu with Stir-Fried Vegetables and Brown Rice

Day 23:

- **Breakfast:**

    - o **Option 1:** Smoothie (Spinach, Banana, and Almond Milk)

    - o **Option 2:** Oatmeal with Almonds and Dried Cranberries

- **Lunch:**

    - o **Option 1:** Tomato Basil Soup with Whole Grain Bread

    - o **Option 2:** Grilled Chicken Caesar Salad with a Light Dressing

- **Snack:**

    - o **Option 1:** Apple Slices with Peanut Butter

    - o **Option 2:** Handful of Trail Mix (Nuts, Seeds, and Dried Fruits)

- **Dinner:**

    - o **Option 1:** Grilled Turkey Burgers with Sweet Potato Fries

    - o **Option 2:** Zucchini Noodles with Marinara Sauce and Grilled Shrimp

Day 24:

- **Breakfast:**

    - o **Option 1:** Greek Yogurt with Honey, Granola, and Mixed Berries

    - o **Option 2:** Scrambled Eggs with Avocado and Whole Grain Toast

- **Lunch:**

    - o **Option 1:** Lentil Salad with Cucumber, Tomatoes, and Feta

    - o **Option 2:** Quinoa Bowl with Black Beans, Corn, and Avocado

- **Snack:**

    - o **Option 1:** Carrot Sticks with Hummus

    - o **Option 2:** Celery Sticks with Almond Butter

- **Dinner:**

    - o **Option 1:** Grilled Chicken Breast with Brown Rice and Steamed Green Beans

    - o **Option 2:** Baked Tilapia with Garlic and Lemon, served with Asparagus

Day 25:

- **Breakfast:**

    - o **Option 1:** Smoothie Bowl with Banana, Blueberries, and Flaxseeds

    - o **Option 2:** Whole Grain Pancakes with Maple Syrup and Fresh Berries

- **Lunch:**

    - o **Option 1:** Spinach and Chickpea Salad with Olive Oil Dressing

    - o **Option 2:** Tomato Basil Soup with Whole Grain Crackers

- **Snack:**

  - o **Option 1:** Mixed Fruit Salad

  - o **Option 2:** Sliced Bell Peppers with Guacamole

- **Dinner:**

  - o **Option 1:** Baked Salmon with Sweet Potato Fries and a Side Salad

  - o **Option 2:** Turkey Meatballs with Marinara Sauce and Whole Grain Pasta

Day 26:

- **Breakfast:**

  - o **Option 1:** Smoothie (Kale, Mango, and Coconut Water)

  - o **Option 2:** Overnight Oats with Almond Butter and Chia Seeds

- **Lunch:**

  - o **Option 1:** Avocado and Cucumber Sushi Rolls

  - o **Option 2:** Grilled Vegetable Wrap with Hummus

- **Snack:**

    o **Option 1:** Handful of Mixed Nuts

    o **Option 2:** Apple Slices with Peanut Butter

- **Dinner:**

    o **Option 1:** Grilled Chicken with Roasted Brussels Sprouts

    o **Option 2:** Baked Cod with Garlic, Lemon, and a Side of Asparagus

Day 27:

- **Breakfast:**

    o **Option 1:** Whole Grain Cereal with Almond Milk and Sliced Bananas

    o **Option 2:** Smoothie (Blueberries, Banana, Spinach, and Almond Milk)

- **Lunch:**

    o **Option 1:** Lentil Soup with Whole Grain Bread

    o **Option 2:** Greek Salad with Grilled Chicken

- **Snack:**

    - o **Option 1:** Celery Sticks with Almond Butter

    - o **Option 2:** Sliced Cucumber with Cottage Cheese

- **Dinner:**

    - o **Option 1:** Grilled Shrimp with Zucchini Noodles and Pesto

    - o **Option 2:** Grilled Turkey Burgers with Sweet Potato Fries

Day 28:

- **Breakfast:**

    - o **Option 1:** Chia Pudding with Mixed Berries

    - o **Option 2:** Greek Yogurt with Honey, Granola, and Mixed Berries

- **Lunch:**

  - o **Option 1:** Quinoa Salad with Roasted Vegetables and Feta

  - o **Option 2:** Spinach and Quinoa Salad with Lemon Dressing

- **Snack:**

  - o **Option 1:** Handful of Mixed Nuts

  - o **Option 2:** Sliced Bell Peppers with Guacamole

- **Dinner:**

  - o **Option 1:** Baked Tilapia with Garlic and Lemon, served with Asparagus

  - o **Option 2:** Zucchini Noodles with Marinara Sauce and Grilled Shrimp

---

This concludes the 4-week "Moon Diet" plan, with each week aligned to the phases of the moon and meals designed to be nutritious, affordable, and easy to prepare. Let me know if you need any further adjustments or additional details!

SECOND OPTION LIST

Week 1: New Moon Phase

Focus: Cleansing and detoxifying the body

Day 1:

- **Breakfast:**

    o **Option 1:** Smoothie (Apple, Ginger, Spinach, and Water)

    o **Option 2:** Overnight Chia Pudding with Coconut Milk and Sliced Strawberries

- **Lunch:**

    o **Option 1:** Butternut Squash Soup with a Side of Mixed Greens

    o **Option 2:** Grilled Vegetable and Hummus Wrap

- **Snack:**

    - o **Option 1:** Sliced Pear with Almond Butter

    - o **Option 2:** Cucumber and Tomato Salad with Balsamic Vinaigrette

- **Dinner:**

    - o **Option 1:** Steamed Cod with Lemon, Garlic, and Wilted Spinach

    - o **Option 2:** Lentil Stew with Carrots and Celery

Day 2:

- **Breakfast:**

    - o **Option 1:** Smoothie (Pineapple, Kale, and Coconut Water)

    - o **Option 2:** Quinoa Porridge with Almond Milk and Blueberries

- **Lunch:**

    - o **Option 1:** Grilled Chicken with Mixed Green Salad and Olive Oil Dressing

    - o **Option 2:** Tomato and Cucumber Salad with Feta Cheese

- **Snack:**

    o **Option 1:** Bell Pepper Slices with Hummus

    o **Option 2:** Fresh Orange Slices with a Sprinkle of Cinnamon

- **Dinner:**

    o **Option 1:** Baked Eggplant with Tomato and Mozzarella

    o **Option 2:** Roasted Cauliflower with Garlic and Lemon, served with Quinoa

Day 3:

- **Breakfast:**

    o **Option 1:** Oatmeal with Pumpkin Seeds, Cinnamon, and Sliced Apple

    o **Option 2:** Greek Yogurt with Honey, Chia Seeds, and Mixed Berries

- **Lunch:**

    o **Option 1:** Spinach and Quinoa Salad with Diced Avocado and a Lemon Dressing

    o **Option 2:** Zucchini Noodles with Cherry Tomatoes and Pesto

- **Snack:**

    o **Option 1:** Sliced Carrots with Guacamole

    o **Option 2:** Apple Slices with a Sprinkle of Cinnamon

- **Dinner:**

    o **Option 1:** Grilled Salmon with Steamed Green Beans and Brown Rice

    o **Option 2:** Turkey Meatloaf with Sweet Potato Mash

Day 4:

- **Breakfast:**

    o **Option 1:** Smoothie (Banana, Spinach, Almond Butter, and Almond Milk)

    o **Option 2:** Whole Grain Toast with Avocado and Cherry Tomatoes

- **Lunch:**

    o **Option 1:** Grilled Shrimp with Mango Salsa and Mixed Greens

    o **Option 2:** Lentil Salad with Cherry Tomatoes, Cucumber, and Olive Oil

- **Snack:**

    - o **Option 1:** Celery Sticks with Cottage Cheese

    - o **Option 2:** Smoothie (Mango, Pineapple, and Coconut Water)

- **Dinner:**

    - o **Option 1:** Baked Chicken Breast with Roasted Brussels Sprouts

    - o **Option 2:** Grilled Portobello Mushrooms with Quinoa and Steamed Vegetables

Day 5:

- **Breakfast:**

    - o **Option 1:** Smoothie (Mixed Berries, Greek Yogurt, and Almond Milk)

    - o **Option 2:** Chia Seed Pudding with Almond Milk and Fresh Raspberries

- **Lunch:**

  - o **Option 1:** Caprese Salad with Fresh Basil and Balsamic Glaze

  - o **Option 2:** Greek Salad with Grilled Chicken and a Light Olive Oil Dressing

- **Snack:**

  - o **Option 1:** Sliced Cucumber with Hummus

  - o **Option 2:** Mixed Berries with a Sprinkle of Chia Seeds

- **Dinner:**

  - o **Option 1:** Baked Salmon with Sweet Potato Fries and Steamed Asparagus

  - o **Option 2:** Grilled Turkey Breast with Quinoa and Roasted Vegetables

Day 6:

- **Breakfast:**

  - o **Option 1:** Smoothie (Apple, Carrot, Ginger, and Water)

  - o **Option 2:** Whole Grain Cereal with Almond Milk and Sliced Strawberries

- **Lunch:**

  - o **Option 1:** Quinoa and Black Bean Salad with a Lime Dressing

  - o **Option 2:** Grilled Chicken Wrap with Lettuce, Tomato, and Avocado

- **Snack:**

  - o **Option 1:** Sliced Pear with Almond Butter

  - o **Option 2:** Smoothie (Cucumber, Lime, and Mint)

- **Dinner:**

  - o **Option 1:** Grilled Shrimp with Garlic and Lemon, served with Steamed Vegetables

  - o **Option 2:** Stuffed Bell Peppers with Ground Turkey and Brown Rice

Day 7:

- **Breakfast:**

  - o **Option 1:** Smoothie (Banana, Oats, Almond Butter, and Almond Milk)

  - o **Option 2:** Overnight Oats with Blueberries and Chia Seeds

- **Lunch:**

  - o **Option 1:** Tomato Soup with Whole Grain Crackers

  - o **Option 2:** Spinach Salad with Strawberries, Walnuts, and a Balsamic Dressing

- **Snack:**

  - o **Option 1:** Celery Sticks with Almond Butter

  - o **Option 2:** Mixed Fruit Salad with a Honey-Lime Dressing

- **Dinner:**

  - o **Option 1:** Grilled Chicken with Steamed Broccoli and Brown Rice

  - o **Option 2:** Baked Fish with Garlic, Lemon, and a Side of Green Beans

Week 2: Waxing Crescent Moon

Focus: Building and nourishing the body

Day 8:

- **Breakfast:**

    - **Option 1:** Scrambled Eggs with Spinach and Whole Grain Toast

    - **Option 2:** Smoothie (Mixed Berries, Oats, and Almond Milk)

- **Lunch:**

    - **Option 1:** Grilled Chicken Caesar Salad with a Light Dressing

    - **Option 2:** Roasted Vegetable and Quinoa Salad

- **Snack:**

    - **Option 1:** Hard-Boiled Egg with a Sprinkle of Paprika

    - **Option 2:** Mixed Nuts and Dried Cranberries

- **Dinner:**

  - o **Option 1:** Grilled Steak with Roasted Sweet Potatoes and Steamed Broccoli

  - o **Option 2:** Baked Chicken with Wild Rice and Roasted Vegetables

Day 9:

- **Breakfast:**

  - o **Option 1:** Greek Yogurt with Honey, Granola, and Mixed Berries

  - o **Option 2:** Quinoa Porridge with Cinnamon and Apple Slices

- **Lunch:**

  - o **Option 1:** Tuna Salad with Whole Grain Crackers

  - o **Option 2:** Roasted Beet and Goat Cheese Salad

- **Snack:**

  - o **Option 1:** Apple Slices with Almond Butter

  - o **Option 2:** Smoothie (Spinach, Pineapple, and Coconut Water)

- **Dinner:**

    - o **Option 1:** Grilled Shrimp with Zucchini Noodles and Basil Pesto

    - o **Option 2:** Turkey Meatballs with Spaghetti Squash and Marinara Sauce

Day 10:

- **Breakfast:**

    - o **Option 1:** Whole Grain Pancakes with Maple Syrup and Fresh Raspberries

    - o **Option 2:** Smoothie (Banana, Spinach, Almond Butter, and Almond Milk)

- **Lunch:**

    - o **Option 1:** Spinach and Feta Quinoa Salad

    - o **Option 2:** Chicken and Vegetable Stir-fry with Brown Rice

- **Snack:**

  - o **Option 1:** Carrot Sticks with Guacamole

  - o **Option 2:** Pear Slices with Cinnamon

- **Dinner:**

  - o **Option 1:** Grilled Chicken Breast with Wild Rice and Steamed Green Beans

  - o **Option 2:** Baked Cod with Roasted Brussels Sprouts

Day 11:

- **Breakfast:**

  - o **Option 1:** Smoothie (Kale, Pineapple, and Coconut Water)

  - o **Option 2:** Whole Grain Toast with Avocado and Poached Egg

- **Lunch:**

  - o **Option 1:** Lentil Salad with Cucumber, Tomatoes, and Lemon Dressing

  - o **Option 2:** Turkey and Avocado Wrap

- **Snack:**

  - o **Option 1:** Handful of Mixed Nuts

  - o **Option 2:** Cucumber Slices with Cottage Cheese

- **Dinner:**

  - o **Option 1:** Grilled Salmon with Sweet Potato Wedges and a Side Salad

  - o **Option 2:** Tofu Stir-fry with Broccoli and Brown Rice

Day 12:

- **Breakfast:**

  - o **Option 1:** Greek Yogurt with Honey, Granola, and Mixed Berries

  - o **Option 2:** Oatmeal with Almonds and Dried Cranberries

- **Lunch:**

  - o **Option 1:** Grilled Chicken Caesar Salad with a Light Dressing

  - o **Option 2:** Quinoa and Black Bean Salad with Lime Dressing

- **Snack:**

  - o **Option 1:** Celery Sticks with Almond Butter

  - o **Option 2:** Mixed Fruit Salad with Mint

- **Dinner:**

  - o **Option 1:** Grilled Turkey Burgers with Sweet Potato Fries

  - o **Option 2:** Stuffed Bell Peppers with Ground Beef and Brown Rice

Day 13:

- **Breakfast:**

  - o **Option 1:** Smoothie (Banana, Spinach, and Almond Milk)

  - o **Option 2:** Greek Yogurt with Honey and Walnuts

- **Lunch:**

  - o **Option 1:** Black Bean Soup with Whole Grain Crackers

  - o **Option 2:** Greek Salad with Grilled Chicken

- **Snack:**

    o **Option 1:** Bell Pepper Slices with Hummus

    o **Option 2:** Mixed Berries with Almonds

- **Dinner:**

    o **Option 1:** Grilled Chicken with Roasted Brussels Sprouts

    o **Option 2:** Zucchini Noodles with Pesto and Grilled Shrimp

Day 14:

- **Breakfast:**

    o **Option 1:** Smoothie (Blueberries, Banana, Almond Butter, and Almond Milk)

    o **Option 2:** Chia Seed Pudding with Coconut Milk and Fresh Mango

- **Lunch:**

  - o **Option 1:** Caprese Salad with a Drizzle of Balsamic Vinegar

  - o **Option 2:** Lentil and Quinoa Salad with Lemon Dressing

- **Snack:**

  - o **Option 1:** Almonds and Dried Apricots

  - o **Option 2:** Mixed Fruit Salad with a Squeeze of Lime

- **Dinner:**

  - o **Option 1:** Grilled Salmon with Quinoa and Steamed Asparagus

  - o **Option 2:** Grilled Steak with Sweet Potato Mash and a Side Salad

Week 3: Full Moon

Focus: Energy and activity, more substantial meals

Day 15:

- **Breakfast:**

    - **Option 1:** Whole Grain Pancakes with Honey and Fresh Blueberries

    - **Option 2:** Scrambled Eggs with Avocado and Whole Grain Toast

- **Lunch:**

    - **Option 1:** Spinach and Quinoa Salad with Feta Cheese and Olive Oil Dressing

    - **Option 2:** Tuna Salad with Whole Grain Crackers

- **Snack:**

    - **Option 1:** Greek Yogurt with Honey and Almonds

    - **Option 2:** Smoothie (Mixed Berries, Greek Yogurt, and Oats)

- **Dinner:**

  - o **Option 1:** Grilled Chicken Breast with Brown Rice and Steamed Broccoli

  - o **Option 2:** Baked Cod with Garlic, Lemon, and Roasted Asparagus

Day 16:

- **Breakfast:**

  - o **Option 1:** Oatmeal with Almond Butter, Chia Seeds, and Sliced Bananas

  - o **Option 2:** Smoothie (Kale, Pineapple, and Coconut Water)

- **Lunch:**

  - o **Option 1:** Grilled Vegetable Wrap with Hummus

  - o **Option 2:** Tomato Basil Soup with Whole Grain Bread

- **Snack:**

  - o **Option 1:** Apple Slices with Peanut Butter

  - o **Option 2:** Handful of Trail Mix (Nuts, Seeds, and Dried Fruits)

- **Dinner:**

    - o **Option 1:** Grilled Chicken with Steamed Broccoli and Brown Rice

    - o **Option 2:** Baked Fish with Lemon, Garlic, and Roasted Brussels Sprouts

Day 17:

- **Breakfast:**

    - o **Option 1:** Smoothie Bowl with Banana, Blueberries, and Chia Seeds

    - o **Option 2:** Scrambled Eggs with Spinach and Whole Grain Toast

- **Lunch:**

    - o **Option 1:** Greek Salad with Grilled Chicken and Olive Oil Dressing

    - o **Option 2:** Lentil Soup with Whole Grain Crackers

- **Snack:**

    - o **Option 1:** Carrot Sticks with Guacamole

    - o **Option 2:** Apple Slices with Almond Butter

- **Dinner:**

  - o **Option 1:** Grilled Turkey Burgers with Sweet Potato Fries

  - o **Option 2:** Zucchini Noodles with Pesto and Grilled Shrimp

Day 18:

- **Breakfast:**

  - o **Option 1:** Chia Pudding with Coconut Milk and Fresh Berries

  - o **Option 2:** Whole Grain Pancakes with Maple Syrup and Fresh Strawberries

- **Lunch:**

  - o **Option 1:** Spinach Salad with Strawberries, Walnuts, and Balsamic Dressing

  - o **Option 2:** Grilled Chicken Caesar Salad with a Light Dressing

- **Snack:**

  - o **Option 1:** Rice Cakes with Almond Butter and Sliced Bananas

  - o **Option 2:** Mixed Nuts and Dried Cranberries

- **Dinner:**
    - o **Option 1:** Grilled Chicken with Sweet Potato Mash and Steamed Asparagus
    - o **Option 2:** Baked Fish with Lemon, Garlic, and Roasted Brussels Sprouts

Day 19:

- **Breakfast:**
    - o **Option 1:** Smoothie (Spinach, Mango, and Coconut Water)
    - o **Option 2:** Greek Yogurt with Honey, Granola, and Mixed Berries

- **Lunch:**
    - o **Option 1:** Avocado and Cucumber Sushi Rolls
    - o **Option 2:** Quinoa Salad with Roasted Vegetables and Feta Cheese

- **Snack:**
    - o **Option 1:** Apple Slices with Peanut Butter
    - o **Option 2:** Mixed Fruit Salad with a Honey-Lime Dressing

- **Dinner:**

  - o **Option 1:** Grilled Shrimp with Zucchini Noodles and Pesto

  - o **Option 2:** Turkey Meatballs with Spaghetti Squash and Marinara Sauce

Day 20:

- **Breakfast:**

  - o **Option 1:** Smoothie (Banana, Spinach, and Almond Butter)

  - o **Option 2:** Overnight Oats with Almond Milk and Chia Seeds

- **Lunch:**

  - o **Option 1:** Tuna Salad with Whole Grain Crackers

  - o **Option 2:** Spinach and Quinoa Salad with Lemon Dressing

- **Snack:**

  - o **Option 1:** Sliced Cucumber with Cottage Cheese

  - o **Option 2:** Celery Sticks with Almond Butter

- **Dinner:**

  - o **Option 1:** Baked Tilapia with Garlic, Lemon, and a Side of Green Beans

  - o **Option 2:** Grilled Chicken with Roasted Sweet Potatoes and Steamed Broccoli

Day 21:

- **Breakfast:**

  - o **Option 1:** Whole Grain Cereal with Almond Milk and Sliced Bananas

  - o **Option 2:** Smoothie (Blueberries, Banana, and Almond Butter)

- **Lunch:**

  - o **Option 1:** Spinach and Chickpea Salad with a Lemon Dressing

  - o **Option 2:** Tomato Basil Soup with Whole Grain Crackers

- **Snack:**

  - o **Option 1:** Hard-Boiled Egg with a Sprinkle of Paprika

  - o **Option 2:** Mixed Nuts and Dried Fruit

- **Dinner:**

    - o **Option 1:** Grilled Steak with Quinoa and Roasted Vegetables

    - o **Option 2:** Stuffed Bell Peppers with Ground Turkey and Brown Rice

Week 4: Waning Crescent Moon

Focus: Preparing for the next cycle, lighter meals

Day 22:

- **Breakfast:**

    - o **Option 1:** Chia Pudding with Coconut Milk and Fresh Berries

    - o **Option 2:** Greek Yogurt with Honey and Walnuts

- **Lunch:**

    - o **Option 1:** Caprese Salad with Fresh Basil and a Balsamic Glaze

    - o **Option 2:** Spinach and Quinoa Salad with Feta Cheese and Olive Oil Dressing

- **Snack:**

    - o **Option 1:** Celery Sticks with Almond Butter

    - o **Option 2:** Mixed Fruit Salad with a Honey-Lime Dressing

- **Dinner:**

    - o **Option 1:** Baked Cod with Lemon and Garlic, served with Steamed Broccoli

    - o **Option 2:** Grilled Tofu with Stir-Fried Vegetables and Brown Rice

Day 23:

- **Breakfast:**

    - o **Option 1:** Smoothie (Spinach, Pineapple, and Coconut Water)

    - o **Option 2:** Whole Grain Oatmeal with Almond Butter and Sliced Bananas

- **Lunch:**

    - o **Option 1:** Tomato Basil Soup with Whole Grain Crackers

    - o **Option 2:** Grilled Chicken Caesar Salad with a Light Dressing

- **Snack:**

  - o **Option 1:** Sliced Pear with Almond Butter

  - o **Option 2:** Celery Sticks with Hummus

- **Dinner:**

  - o **Option 1:** Grilled Turkey Burgers with Sweet Potato Fries

  - o **Option 2:** Zucchini Noodles with Pesto and Grilled Shrimp

Day 24:

- **Breakfast:**

  - o **Option 1:** Greek Yogurt with Honey, Granola, and Mixed Berries

  - o **Option 2:** Scrambled Eggs with Spinach and Whole Grain Toast

- **Lunch:**

  - o **Option 1:** Lentil Salad with Cucumber, Tomatoes, and Feta Cheese

  - o **Option 2:** Grilled Chicken Wrap with Avocado and Tomato

- **Snack:**

  - o **Option 1:** Bell Pepper Slices with Hummus

  - o **Option 2:** Mixed Berries with Almonds

- **Dinner:**

  - o **Option 1:** Grilled Chicken Breast with Wild Rice and Steamed Broccoli

  - o **Option 2:** Baked Tilapia with Garlic, Lemon, and Roasted Asparagus

Day 25:

- **Breakfast:**

  - o **Option 1:** Smoothie Bowl with Banana, Blueberries, and Chia Seeds

  - o **Option 2:** Whole Grain Pancakes with Maple Syrup and Fresh Raspberries

- **Lunch:**

  - o **Option 1:** Spinach and Chickpea Salad with Olive Oil Dressing

  - o **Option 2:** Tomato Basil Soup with Whole Grain Crackers

- **Snack:**

    o **Option 1:** Apple Slices with Almond Butter

    o **Option 2:** Mixed Nuts and Dried Fruit

- **Dinner:**

    o **Option 1:** Baked Salmon with Sweet Potato Fries and Steamed Asparagus

    o **Option 2:** Turkey Meatballs with Spaghetti Squash and Marinara Sauce

Day 26:

- **Breakfast:**

    o **Option 1:** Smoothie (Kale, Mango, and Coconut Water)

    o **Option 2:** Overnight Oats with Almond Milk and Chia Seeds

- **Lunch:**

    o **Option 1:** Avocado and Cucumber Sushi Rolls

    o **Option 2:** Grilled Chicken Caesar Salad with a Light Dressing

- **Snack:**

  - Option 1: Sliced Bell Peppers with Hummus

  - Option 2: Celery Sticks with Almond Butter

- **Dinner:**

  - Option 1: Grilled Chicken with Roasted Brussels Sprouts

  - Option 2: Baked Cod with Lemon and Garlic, served with Steamed Green Beans

Day 27:

- **Breakfast:**

  - Option 1: Whole Grain Cereal with Almond Milk and Sliced Bananas

  - Option 2: Smoothie (Blueberries, Banana, and Almond Butter)

- **Lunch:**

  - Option 1: Lentil Soup with Whole Grain Crackers

  - Option 2: Greek Salad with Grilled Chicken

- **Snack:**

  - o **Option 1:** Carrot Sticks with Guacamole

  - o **Option 2:** Mixed Fruit Salad with a Honey-Lime Dressing

- **Dinner:**

  - o **Option 1:** Grilled Shrimp with Zucchini Noodles and Pesto

  - o **Option 2:** Grilled Turkey Burgers with Sweet Potato Fries

Day 28:

- **Breakfast:**

  - o **Option 1:** Chia Pudding with Coconut Milk and Fresh Strawberries

  - o **Option 2:** Greek Yogurt with Honey, Granola, and Mixed Berries

- **Lunch:**

  - o **Option 1:** Quinoa Salad with Roasted Vegetables and Feta Cheese

  - o **Option 2:** Spinach and Quinoa Salad with Lemon Dressing

- **Snack:**

  - o **Option 1:** Mixed Nuts and Dried Cranberries

  - o **Option 2:** Sliced Cucumber with Cottage Cheese

- **Dinner:**

  - o **Option 1:** Baked Tilapia with Garlic and Lemon, served with Roasted Asparagus

  - o **Option 2:** Zucchini Noodles with Pesto and Grilled Shrimp

EXTRA – NUTS, the best part!!

1. Almonds

Benefits:

- **High in Vitamin E:** Almonds are rich in vitamin E, an antioxidant that helps protect your cells from oxidative damage.

- **Heart Health:** They contain healthy fats that can help reduce bad cholesterol levels and lower the risk of heart disease.

- **Weight Management:** Almonds are high in fiber and protein, which can help keep you feeling full and reduce overall calorie intake.

2. Walnuts

Benefits:

- **Rich in Omega-3 Fatty Acids:** Walnuts are an excellent source of plant-based omega-3s, which are crucial for brain health and reducing inflammation.

- **Antioxidant Properties:** They contain powerful antioxidants that can help fight oxidative stress and inflammation in the body.

- **Heart Health:** Regular consumption of walnuts has been linked to improved heart health and reduced cholesterol levels.

3. Cashews

Benefits:

- **High in Magnesium:** Cashews provide a good amount of magnesium, which is important for energy production, bone health, and muscle relaxation.

- **Heart Health:** They contain heart-healthy monounsaturated fats that can support cardiovascular health.

- **Rich in Copper:** Cashews are a good source of copper, which is essential for iron metabolism, immune function, and maintaining healthy skin.

4. Pistachios

Benefits:

- **High in Protein:** Pistachios are one of the most protein-rich nuts, making them a great

- option for those looking to increase their protein intake.

- **Rich in Antioxidants:** They contain lutein and zeaxanthin, antioxidants that support eye health.

- **Weight Management:** Pistachios are low in calories compared to other nuts and are high in fiber, which can help with satiety and weight control.

5. Brazil Nuts

Benefits:

- **Rich in Selenium:** Brazil nuts are one of the best dietary sources of selenium, a mineral that plays a key role in thyroid function and antioxidant defense.

- **Heart Health:** The healthy fats in Brazil nuts support heart health, and their selenium content helps reduce inflammation.

- **Immune Support:** Selenium in Brazil nuts is also important for a healthy immune system.

6. Hazelnuts

Benefits:

- **High in Vitamin E:** Like almonds, hazelnuts are rich in vitamin E, which supports skin health and acts as an antioxidant.

- **Supports Heart Health:** Hazelnuts contain monounsaturated fats and other nutrients that help reduce the risk of cardiovascular disease.

- **Brain Health:** The high levels of folate and manganese in hazelnuts are beneficial for brain function and cognitive health.

7. Pecans

Benefits:

- **Rich in Antioxidants:** Pecans have a high antioxidant content, which can help protect against oxidative stress and chronic diseases.

- **Heart Health:** The monounsaturated fats in pecans support heart health by lowering bad cholesterol levels.

- **Weight Management:** Pecans are satisfying and nutrient-dense, which can help with weight management when eaten in moderation.

8. Macadamia Nuts

Benefits:

- **High in Healthy Fats:** Macadamia nuts are rich in monounsaturated fats, which are beneficial for heart health and reducing inflammation.

- **Supports Brain Health:** The healthy fats and antioxidants in macadamia nuts may help protect the brain and support cognitive function.

- **Rich in Manganese:** Macadamia nuts provide a good amount of manganese, which is important for bone health and metabolism.

9. Pine Nuts

Benefits:

- **Rich in Vitamins and Minerals:** Pine nuts are a good source of vitamins E and K, magnesium, and zinc.

- **Appetite Control:** Pine nuts contain pinolenic acid, which has been shown to promote the release of hunger-suppressing hormones.

- **Heart Health:** The healthy fats in pine nuts can help improve cholesterol levels and support heart health.

10. Peanuts

Benefits:

- **High in Protein:** Peanuts are a great source of plant-based protein, making them an excellent option for muscle repair and growth.

- **Rich in Niacin:** Peanuts provide a significant amount of niacin (vitamin B3), which supports brain health and reduces the risk of Alzheimer's disease.

- **Antioxidant Properties:** Peanuts contain resveratrol, an antioxidant also found in red wine, which has been linked to various health benefits, including heart health.

11. Pumpkin Seeds

Benefits:

- **Rich in Magnesium:** Pumpkin seeds are one of the best natural sources of magnesium, which is crucial for energy production, muscle function, and bone health.

- **High in Zinc:** They are an excellent source of zinc, which supports immune function, skin health, and reproductive health.

- **Antioxidant Properties:** Pumpkin seeds contain a variety of antioxidants, which can help reduce inflammation and protect cells from oxidative damage.

- **Heart Health:** The healthy fats, magnesium, and antioxidants in pumpkin seeds contribute to heart health by improving cholesterol levels and reducing blood pressure.

General Tips:

- **Portion Control:** Nuts and seeds are calorie-dense, so it is important to enjoy them in moderation. A handful (about 1 ounce or 28 grams) is a good serving size.

- **Variety:** Incorporating a variety of nuts and seeds into your diet ensures you get a broad range of nutrients.

- **Unsalted and Raw:** Choose unsalted and raw or dry-roasted nuts and seeds to avoid added sodium and unhealthy fats.

Here's a list of foods, snacks, and drinks to <u>avoid</u> during the 4-week "Moon Diet" period to help you stay on track with your goals.

Foods to Avoid:

1. **Processed Foods:**

   o   Packaged snacks like chips, crackers, and cookies

   o   Ready-made meals, frozen dinners, and instant noodles

   o   Fast food items (burgers, fries, pizzas)

2. **Sugary Foods:**

   o   Candy, chocolate bars, and sweets

   o   Sugary cereals and granola bars

   o   Desserts like cakes, pastries, and doughnuts

   o   Ice cream and frozen desserts

Refined Carbohydrates:

- o White bread, white rice, and regular pasta

- o Pastries, muffins, and white flour-based baked goods

3. **Fried Foods:**

- o Deep-fried snacks like French fries, fried chicken, and doughnuts

- o Tempura or batter-fried foods

4. **High-Sodium Foods:**

- o Canned soups and vegetables with added salt

- o Processed meats like sausages, bacon, and deli meats

- o Packaged sauces, condiments, and seasoning mixes with high sodium content

5. **Red and Processed Meats:**

- o Sausages, bacon, hot dogs, and other processed meats

- o High-fat cuts of beef, lamb, and pork

6. **Dairy Products (High fat):**

   o   Full-fat milk, cream, and high-fat cheeses

   o   Butter and heavy cream-based sauces

7. **Artificial Sweeteners:**

   o   Diet sodas, sugar-free candies, and desserts

   o   Artificially sweetened snacks and beverages

Snacks to Avoid:

1. **Sugary Snacks:**

   o   Candy, chocolate, and other sweets

   o   Sugary granola bars and snack cakes

2. **High-Calorie, Low-Nutrient Snacks:**

   o   Potato chips, cheese puffs, and other salty snacks

   o   Packaged cookies, cakes, and pastries

3. **Processed Nut Butters:**

   o   Peanut butter with added sugars and hydrogenated oils

   o   Flavored nut spreads with added sugars

4. **Sugary Yogurts:**

   o   Flavored yogurts with added sugars

   o   Yogurt desserts and parfaits with added sugars

Drinks to Avoid:

1. **Sugary Beverages:**

   o   Soda and sugary soft drinks

   o   Energy drinks and sports drinks with high sugar content

   o   Sweetened iced teas and lemonades

2. **Alcohol:**

   o   Beer, wine, and spirits, particularly those with added sugars

   o   Cocktails and mixed drinks with sugary mixers

3. **Caffeinated Beverages (Excessive Amounts):**

   o Coffee and energy drinks in large quantities (limit to 1-2 cups per day if consumed)

   o Sugary lattes, frappes, and other flavored coffee drinks

4. **Fruit Juices (Store-bought, Sweetened):**

   o Packaged fruit juices with added sugars

   o Sweetened fruit drinks and fruit punch

5. **Artificially Sweetened Drinks:**

   o Diet sodas and sugar-free drinks with artificial sweeteners

   o Flavored water with artificial sweeteners

General Tips:

- **Minimize refined sugars:** Look out for hidden sugars in sauces, dressings, and packaged foods.

- **Limit processed grains:** Stick to whole grains like brown rice, quinoa, and oats.

- **Avoid excess salt:** Check labels for sodium content and try to cook more at home where you can control the seasoning.

- **Hydrate with water:** opt for water, herbal teas, and natural detox waters infused with lemon, cucumber, or mint instead of sugary drinks.

By avoiding these items, you'll help maximize the benefits of the "Moon Diet" and support your overall health goals during this 4-week period.

In addition to following the "Moon Diet," incorporating specific activities can enhance weight loss and overall well-being during this 4-week period. Here's a list of activities that can complement your diet:

Physical Activities:

1. **Daily Exercise:**

   o **Cardio Workouts:** Engage in 30-45 minutes of cardio exercises such as brisk walking, jogging, cycling, or swimming. These helps burn calories and improve cardiovascular health.

   o **Strength Training:** Incorporate 2-3 days of strength training per week using bodyweight exercises (e.g.,

- o squats, lunges, push-ups) or light weights. This helps build muscle, which increases metabolism.

- o **High-Intensity Interval Training (HIIT):** Include 1-2 sessions of HIIT per week to boost metabolism and burn fat. These short, intense bursts of exercise followed by rest periods are highly effective.

- o **Yoga or Pilates:** Practice yoga or Pilates 2-3 times per week to improve flexibility, strength, and mindfulness. These activities also help reduce stress, which can aid in weight loss.

2. **Daily Walking:**

- o Aim for at least 10,000 steps per day. Walking is a low-impact way to keep your body moving and increase daily calorie burn.

3. **Stretching:**

   o Incorporate 10-15 minutes of stretching daily, especially after workouts. This improves flexibility, reduces the risk of injury, and promotes muscle recovery.

Mindfulness and Relaxation:

1. **Meditation:**

   o Practice mindfulness meditation for 10-20 minutes daily. Focus on your breath, body, or a guided meditation. Meditation reduces stress, which can prevent stress-related eating and support weight loss.

   o **Lunar Meditation:** Sync your meditation practices with the phases of the moon. For example, during the New Moon, focus on setting intentions and letting go of old habits; during the Full Moon, focus on gratitude and reflection.

2. **Deep Breathing Exercises:**

   o   Practice deep breathing techniques (e.g., diaphragmatic breathing) for 5-10 minutes daily. This can help manage stress, improve focus, and support your weight loss journey.

3. **Calm Music and Sound Therapy:**

   o   Listen to calming music, nature sounds, or binaural beats to relax and reduce stress. Consider listening to this music while meditating, doing yoga, or before bedtime to improve sleep quality.

4. **Visualization:**

   o   Spend a few minutes each day visualizing your weight loss goals. Imagine yourself achieving your desired weight, feeling healthy, and confident. Visualization can reinforce positive behaviors and keep you motivated.

Sleep and Recovery:

1. **Prioritize Sleep:**

   o   Aim for 7-9 hours of quality sleep each night. Poor sleep can disrupt hormones that regulate hunger and appetite, making weight loss more challenging.

   o   Create a relaxing bedtime routine, such as reading a book, listening to calm music, or taking a warm bath before bed.

2. **Power Naps:**

   o   Take short naps (15-30 minutes) if needed during the day to recharge and reduce fatigue.

3. **Digital Detox Before Bedtime:**

   o   Avoid screens (phones, tablets, computers) at least an hour before bed. The blue light emitted by screens can interfere with your sleep cycle.

Hydration and Detox:

1. **Stay Hydrated:**

   o Drink at least 8 glasses of water per day. Staying hydrated supports metabolism and helps control hunger.

   o Consider drinking herbal teas (like green tea, peppermint tea, or chamomile tea) to promote relaxation and digestion.

2. **Detoxifying Drinks:**

   o Start your day with a glass of warm lemon water to kickstart your metabolism and aid digestion.

   o Incorporate detoxifying drinks such as cucumber and mint-infused water, or apple cider vinegar diluted in water before meals.

Lifestyle Adjustments:

1. **Mindful Eating:**

   o Practice mindful eating by paying attention to hunger cues, eating slowly, and savoring each bite. This can help prevent overeating and improve digestion.

   o Avoid distractions (e.g., TV, phone) during meals to stay focused on your food.

2. **Journaling:**

   o Keep a journal to track your meals, exercise, thoughts, and feelings. Journaling can help you stay accountable, identify patterns, and make necessary adjustments.

3. **Sunlight Exposure:**

   o Spend time outdoors in natural sunlight each day. Sunlight helps regulate your circadian rhythm, supports vitamin D production, and can boost mood and energy levels.

4. **Social Support:**

    o Surround yourself with supportive friends or join a group that shares similar health goals. Having a support system can keep you motivated and accountable.

Stress Management:

1. **Aromatherapy:**

    o Use essential oils like lavender, eucalyptus, or chamomile in a diffuser to create a calming environment. Aromatherapy can help reduce stress and improve sleep quality.

2. **Hot Baths or Showers:**

    o Take warm baths or showers to relax your muscles and mind. Add Epsom salts to your bath to soothe sore muscles and detoxify your body.

By integrating these activities with your diet, you can optimize your weight loss journey and promote a balanced, healthy lifestyle.

Here are 20 artists and sources where you can find calm, meditation, and relaxation music to support your journey:

Artists and Composers:

1. **Steven Halpern** - A pioneer in sound healing, known for his relaxing, meditative compositions.

2. **Deuter** - German composer known for his meditative and ambient music, often featuring flutes and nature sounds.

3. **Liquid Mind** - A project by Chuck Wild, creating deeply relaxing, tranquil music perfect for meditation.

4. **Brian Eno** - Known for his ambient music, including the famous album "Ambient 1: Music for Airports."

5. **Enya** - Irish singer known for her ethereal, soothing music, blending Celtic and New Age influences.

6. **Llewellyn** - British composer known for his meditation, healing, and relaxation music, often inspired by nature.

7.

8. **Anugama** - German musician who creates soothing, spiritual music ideal for meditation and relaxation.

9. **Sacred Earth** - Australian duo that creates beautiful, meditative music with an emphasis on spirituality and healing.

10. **Ananda Giri** - Composer of spiritual and meditative music, often used in mindfulness and meditation practices.

11. **Tenzin Choegyal** - Tibetan musician blending traditional Tibetan music with modern meditative sounds.

12. **George Winston** - American pianist known for his peaceful, reflective solo piano works.

13. **Yiruma** - South Korean pianist and composer known for his serene, calming piano pieces.

14. **Snatam Kaur** - American singer known for her spiritual music, blending Sikh mantras with soothing melodies.

15. **Marconi Union** - British musical trio known for their ambient track "Weightless," which is often cited as one of the most relaxing songs ever.

16. **Kitaro** - Japanese composer and musician, known for his blend of traditional Japanese music with ambient and New Age elements.

17. **Paul Horn** - Flautist known for his "Inside" series of albums, recorded in acoustically rich environments, ideal for meditation.

18. **Laraaji** - American musician and laughter meditation practitioner, known for his ambient and spiritual music.

19. **Moby** - American musician who has released several albums of ambient and meditative music, such as "Long Ambients 1: Calm. Sleep."

20. **Karunesh** - German-born composer known for his fusion of world music, New Age, and meditative sounds.

21. **Kevin Kern** - American pianist known for his gentle, melodic compositions, perfect for relaxation and meditation.

Places to Find Meditation and Relaxation Music:

1. **YouTube:**

   o   Search for channels like "Yellow Brick Cinema," "Meditative Mind," "Calm Radio," and "The Honest Guys" for a wide variety of meditation and relaxation music.

2. **Spotify:**

   o   Explore playlists such as "Peaceful Meditation," "Calm Vibes," "Deep Sleep," and "Relax & Unwind." Many of the artists listed above have dedicated playlists or albums available.

3. **Apple Music:**

   o   Search for curated playlists like "Meditation Essentials," "Yoga & Meditation," and "Ambient Chill."

4. **Pandora:**

   o   Create a custom station based on any of the artists mentioned above or o   search for stations like "Ambient Meditations" and "Relaxation Radio."

5. **Calm App:**

   o   The Calm app offers a wide range of relaxation and meditation music, as well as guided meditations and sleep stories.

6. **Insight Timer:**

   o   This app offers a vast library of free meditation music, guided meditations, and courses from various teachers and composers.

7. **Headspace:**

   o   The Headspace app provides calming music, soundscapes, and guided meditations designed to help you relax and focus.

8. **SoundCloud:**

   o   Search for meditation and ambient music by independent artists. Many meditation teachers and musicians share their work on this platform.

9. **Bandcamp:**

    o   Explore independent artists who specialize in meditation, ambient, and New Age music. You can often purchase and download high-quality tracks directly from the artist.

10. **Amazon Music:**

    o   Search for meditation and relaxation playlists, albums by the artists mentioned, or browse categories like "New Age," "Ambient," and "Instrumental."

These artists and platforms offer a wide range of relaxing music that can enhance your meditation, yoga, or relaxation practices during the "Moon Diet" period.

In addition to following the "Moon Diet," incorporating specific activities can **enhance weight loss and overall well-being during this 4-week period.**

Estimating the cost of all the ingredients for the "Moon Diet" will vary depending on your location, the specific brands you choose, and where you shop. However, I can give you a rough estimate for a typical weekly grocery list based on average prices. Below is a general breakdown of the cost for common items you'll need over the 4 weeks. Prices are based on typical U.S. grocery store averages.

Estimated Weekly Grocery Costs

Fresh Produce:

- **Spinach (1 lb):** $3.00

- **Kale (1 bunch):** $2.50

- **Mixed Greens (1 lb):** $4.00

- **Avocados (4):** $5.00

- **Tomatoes (4):** $4.00

- **Cucumbers (3):** $3.00

- **Bell Peppers (4):** $4.00

- **Broccoli (2 heads):** $3.50

- **Zucchini (4):** $4.00

- **Sweet Potatoes (3):** $3.50

- **Bananas (6):** $2.00

- **Blueberries (1 pint):** $4.00

- **Strawberries (1 lb):** $3.50

- **Apples (6):** $5.00

- **Oranges (6):** $5.00

- **Lemons (4):** $3.00

Proteins:

- **Chicken Breasts (4 lbs):** $16.00

- **Ground Turkey (2 lbs):** $10.00

- **Salmon Fillets (2 lbs):** $20.00

- **Tilapia Fillets (2 lbs):** $12.00

- **Shrimp (2 lbs):** $16.00

- **Tofu (4 blocks):** $8.00

- **Greek Yogurt (32 oz):** $5.00

- **Eggs (1 dozen):** $3.00

- **Canned Tuna (4 cans):** $6.00

- **Lentils (1 lb):** $2.00

- **Chickpeas (4 cans):** $4.00

- **Quinoa (1 lb):** $6.00

Grains and Legumes:

- **Brown Rice (2 lbs):** $4.00

- **Whole Grain Bread (1 loaf):** $3.50

- **Oatmeal (2 lbs):** $3.00

- **Whole Grain Pasta (2 lbs):** $4.00

Dairy and Dairy Alternatives:

- **Almond Milk (1 gallon):** $3.50

- **Cheese (Feta, Goat, Mozzarella – 1 lb total):** $8.00

- **Cottage Cheese (32 oz):** $4.00

Nuts, Seeds, and Healthy Fats:

- **Almonds (1 lb):** $8.00

- **Peanut Butter (16 oz):** $3.00

- **Chia Seeds (8 oz):** $6.00

- **Olive Oil (16 oz):** $6.00

Herbs, Spices, and Condiments:

- **Fresh Herbs (Parsley, Basil – 2 bunches):** $4.00

- **Garlic (1 bulb):** $1.00

- **Ginger (1 root):** $2.00

- **Lemon Juice (1 bottle):** $2.50

Snacks:

- **Mixed Nuts (1 lb):** $8.00

- **Dried Fruits (8 oz):** $4.00

- **Rice Cakes (1 package):** $3.00

Total Estimated Weekly Cost:

- **Weekly Total:** $150 - $180

Total Estimated Monthly Cost:

- **Monthly Total:** $600 - $720

Cost-Saving Tips:

1. **Buy in Bulk:** Purchase items like rice, quinoa, nuts, and seeds in bulk to reduce costs.

2. **Shop Sales:** Look for sales and discounts on meat, fish, and produce. Stock up on non-perishable items when they are on sale.

3. **Seasonal Produce:** Choose seasonal fruits and vegetables to lower costs. For example, strawberries may be cheaper in summer.

4. **Store Brands:** Opt for store-brand items instead of name brands to save money.

5. **Frozen Produce:** Buy frozen fruits and vegetables, which are often cheaper and last longer without compromising nutrition.

6. **Farmers' Markets:** Shop at local farmers' markets for fresh, often cheaper produce, and support local growers.

This rough estimate should give you a good idea of the overall cost. Adjustments can be made based on your location, dietary preferences, and availability of certain items.

Finding the Next Lunar Phases Online

Understanding and keeping track of lunar phases is essential for anyone following the Moon Diet. Here are several reliable ways your readers can easily find the next lunar phases online:

1. Dedicated Lunar Phase Websites

Time and Date (timeanddate.com): This website offers a comprehensive lunar calendar, showing the current phase of the moon and the dates of upcoming phases. Users can select their location to get accurate local lunar information.

Moon Giant (moongiant.com): Moon Giant provides detailed lunar phase data, including the exact times of the new moon, first quarter, full moon, and last quarter phases. The website also includes additional lunar information and trivia.

Lunaf (lunaf.com): Lunaf offers a user-friendly lunar calendar that displays the phases of the moon for each day. The site includes visuals and descriptions, making it easy to understand the lunar cycle.

2. Astronomy and Science Websites

NASA (nasa.gov): NASA's website includes detailed astronomical data, including lunar phases. They often have articles and educational materials about the moon and its phases.

Astronomy.com: This site provides a monthly lunar calendar, and articles related to lunar phases and other celestial events. It's a great resource for anyone interested in astronomy and the moon.

3. Mobile Apps

Moon Phase Calendar & Widget: This app provides an easy-to-use lunar calendar, showing the phases of the moon and offering notifications for significant lunar events. It's available for both iOS and Android devices.

Deluxe Moon: Deluxe Moon is a comprehensive moon app that provides detailed information about the lunar phases, moonrise and moonset times, and much more. It's available on multiple platforms.

My Moon Phase: My Moon Phase is a user-friendly app that shows the current moon phase and provides dates for upcoming phases. It's available for iOS and Android devices.

Search Engines

Google Search: Simply typing "current moon phase" or "next lunar phases" into Google will provide the current moon phase and upcoming phases. Google also displays a small graphic showing the moon's phase.

Bing Search: Like Google, Bing can provide quick information about the current lunar phase and upcoming phases with a simple search query.

5. Social Media and Forums

Reddit: Subreddits like r/astronomy and r/moon often discuss lunar phases and upcoming celestial events. Users can ask questions and get information from the community.

Facebook Groups: There are various Facebook groups dedicated to moon enthusiasts and astronomy, where members share information about lunar phases and related topics.

6. Online Calendars and Widgets

Google Calendar: Users can add lunar phases to their Google Calendar by subscribing to lunar phase calendars available online. This integration allows users to see lunar phases alongside their personal events.

iCal Lunar Phase Calendar: For iPhone users, adding a lunar phase calendar to iCal is simple. Many websites offer downloadable .ics files that can be imported into iCal to keep track of the moon phases.

By using these resources, you can easily stay informed about the lunar phases, making it convenient to follow the Moon Diet effectively. These tools provide accurate and up-to-date information, ensuring that you can align your dietary practices with the lunar cycle.

Thank you for reading and following the steps to achieve a healthier mind and body. Your commitment to well-being is truly inspiring. Stay well!

www.ingramcontent.com/pod-product-compliance
Lightning Source LLC
Chambersburg PA
CBHW071043250726
48653CB00005B/1981